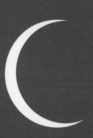

Ten Natural Ways to a Good Night's

sleep

Ten Natural Ways to a Good Night's

sleep

NIKOS LINARDAKIS, M.D.
WITH CARLI DIXON

Gibbs Smith, Publisher
TO ENRICH AND INSPIRE HUMANKIND
Salt Lake City | Charleston | Santa Fe | Santa Barbara

T 100552

FIRST EDITION
11 10 09 08 07   5 4 3 2 1

Published by
Gibbs Smith, Publisher
P.O. Box 667
Layton, Utah 84041

Orders: 1.800.835.4993
www.gibbs-smith.com

Designed by Sterling Hill Productions
Printed and bound in Canada

Library of Congress Cataloging-in-Publication Data
Linardakis, Nikos M.
  Ten natural ways to a good night's sleep / Nikos Linardakis, with Carli Dixon. — 1st ed.
    p. cm.
  ISBN-13: 978-1-4236-0288-0
  ISBN-10: 1-4236-0288-9
  1. Sleep disorders—Popular works. I. Dixon, Carli. II. Title.

RC547.L54 2007
616.8'498—dc22
                        2007027935

Preface

The natural sleep you had as a child is the sleep you deserve and can have again. Natural sleep is safe and effective sleep. Observe a baby sleeping and you will immediately understand this.

Through simple training exercises and natural approaches to sleep, you will learn how to restore healthy sleep to your life by the end of this book. The material in this book can have a profound effect on getting you closer to that deep, natural, restful "baby sleep."

I've wanted to publish this book for several years now. It represents my past fifteen years of work, in which I have been deeply involved in finding ways to help the millions of people suffering from sleep problems.

The story begins in 1987 with graduate and medical school demands. I now realize that I spent over seven years of my life in a sleepless daze! I had to be alert for morning rounds and make difficult decisions at three o'clock in the morning—all with a cup of coffee or a stimulating soda in my hand. The glowing green soda pop was my favorite, and I was addicted. Vending machines were my main source of nutrition.

In 1992, as a doctor in training at Cook County Hospital in Chicago, I could only wrestle in two or three hours of sleep every day. The clinical effects on my mind and body were devastating. Two weeks after I got married, I received the terrifying news that I had developed a primary form of colon cancer and would have to have surgery and follow-up visits for the next three years. Because of my sleep deprivation, I also had glucose deficiency, my immune system crashed, and I developed life-threatening pneumonia. Simply put: I had overworked myself.

What was my solution for better health? I finally took the time to sleep. I spent a lot of money on a nice, comfortable, and supportive bed, and it became my very good friend. I purchased soothing cotton sheets with the finest thread count ever made. I listened to my wife and my mother, who forced me to eat nutritious food again (which I hadn't done in years), and relaxed by reading books. By sleeping well and getting the right nutrition, I recovered fully.

What happened after this turned my life around. My curiosity about sleep and its effect on the health of the body was intense. I became obsessed with understanding sleep studies, and I read everything about sleep. I joined a research team in Chicago studying *jactatio nocturnus*, a rhythmic movement disorder in which children rock in bed and crash their heads and bodies against the walls to help themselves fall asleep. I worked with a pioneer research physician named Dr. Alexander Golbin to help find a solution for these children. With the help of NASA, he invented a rhythmic bed that would rock the child to sleep according to certain patterns in their brain. With a few treatments on the bed rocker, many were helped.

Perhaps it seems an obvious concept now, but back then it was novel: sleep disorders can cause disease, and disease can cause sleep disorders. As a physician I knew this, but I was not listening to my own advice.

In 1994, the study of sleep started to develop in the medical field. Several major universities announced sleep medicine as a course of residency. Case studies began to be published.

In 2003, I started a company for the extraction of natural ingredients to benefit health. We developed a natural sleep dietary supplement using an evidence-based approach founded on clinical studies. This achievement led to winning the Alive Award Silver Medal for best new natural product in 2006.

In this book I will mention the generic pharmaceutical name or the ingredients of natural supplements to inform and educate. No one should become dependent on drugs, form addictions, or become tolerant to products.

My education at the Chicago Medical School included a background in physiology. Studying medicine was a wonderful experience for me; I loved my colleagues, I loved the scientific environment, and I loved learning how the body works. Beneath our skin there are vessels, muscles, nerves, and millions of cells that work in symphony to create a living body—all coordinated by a complex mind. I have a passion for medicine and research, and as a result I have enjoyed the opportunity to speak and lecture at major universities and provide interviews to many media outlets, including NBC, CBS, and the Discovery Channel, and I have published nearly a dozen medical textbooks in pharmacology, pathology, microbiology, and other "ologies."

I no longer have sleep problems because I have discovered the tools to get a good night's sleep—naturally. I've cured *my* inability to sleep. Now it's time for *you* to learn how to do the same.

Please visit www.DrNikos.com to keep me posted on your health and to read about other problems and their solutions.

With appreciation and friendship, yours in health,

Nikos M. Linardakis, M.D.

"Dr. Nikos"

Introduction

We live in a sleep-deprived culture. A recent Gallup poll concludes that 49 percent of Americans say they are suffering from insomnia or sleep-related disorders. Being deprived of sufficient sleep can result in physical exhaustion, irritability, anger, emotional outbursts, poor job performance, headaches, high blood pressure, and accidents.

There are many reasons for sleep deficits, and the purpose of this book is to help you get a good night's sleep using simple, natural, nonprescription methods with proven health benefits.

Before the discovery of fire, people regulated their sleep in relation to natural light and darkness. There was no other choice. After fire, humans discovered oil lamps, and then gas lamps, and then finally—the incandescent lightbulb. Now we can stay awake twenty-four hours a day if we want to. Perhaps we can't blame Thomas Edison for our fast-paced, stressful lifestyle, but today, one-third to one-half of us complain of sleep difficulties.

We either have trouble falling asleep or staying asleep, and we wake up fatigued, not as refreshed and rejuvenated as we would like to be. I stress the drug-free, natural sleep approach because I believe I have discovered a healthy and achievable life-strategy method to getting better sleep. I feel that plant-based supplements may be a part of the solution rather than prescription drugs, which can often have bizarre effects.

There are many reasons why narcotics and hypnotics may not always be the best choice for solving sleep problems. Recently, some of the world's most popular sleep medications have been triggering unusual middle-of-the-night behaviors in users, such as sleep driving, sleep sex, sleep shopping, sleep eating, and even sleep house painting! Some of these activities, such as sleep driving, have become so potentially dangerous that the FDA recently told manufacturers of thirteen sleep medications to put stronger warning labels on their products. For example, users of certain sleep medications have unknowingly driven to the supermarket, taken their truck for a joyride, crashed into parked cars, argued with traffic police, and woken up with broken bones resulting from automobile accidents of which they have no memory. Sleep driving has happened to someone I know personally, and the result was a devastating accident.

In one example of sleep eat-

Helpful Web sites

www.DrNikos.com
www.SleepAndHealth.com
www.apss.org
www.AmericanSleepAssociation.org
www.aasmnet.org
www.SleepApnea.org
www.SleepFoundation.org
www.sleepresearchsociety.org

ing, a British woman mysteriously gained fifty pounds over a seven-month period while taking one sleep medicine. When a family member discovered her asleep in front of her open refrigerator, the mystery was solved.

With more than forty-five million prescriptions for sleep medications written annually, some say that alarming adverse reactions like sleep driving are relatively rare. But I still feel a natural approach is better for many people.

How can you tell if you are getting enough sleep? One sure clue is daytime drowsiness or sleepiness. If you worry that you might fall asleep while driving or nod off every time you sit down in a boring lecture, it's not lunch, monotonous driving, or bad programming that send you nodding off—it's sleep deprivation from the previous night or a series of nights. Otherwise, you might be bored, but you wouldn't fall asleep.

Sleep deprivation is dangerous to your health. University of Chicago researchers have found that skipping sleep can make you old before your time. *Losing sleep can make you old!* I'm stressing this statement because most people are looking for the fountain of youth, and sleep is an important part of maintaining your youthful looks.

If you sleep less than four hours a night, your body may stop regulating hormone levels correctly. There will be a drop in the human growth hormone usually released during sleep, important for youthful growth but also important to repair and rebuild tissue as life goes on. Few classes are taught on healthy sleep in high schools—the time when many of us start burning the candle at both ends and shorting ourselves of the sleep we desperately need for vitality and vigor. Getting enough sleep will help you live a longer, healthier, and more productive life.

Seven or eight hours in restful sleep every night appears to be a healthy norm for most people, an hour or two less than the amount people slept a hundred years ago before the invention of the electric light. Many people need nine hours of sleep to feel completely rested. Athletes in training may need to sleep ten to twelve hours a night, as did the gladiators of old. Your body is unique. You are the best judge of how much sleep is enough.

To find out how much sleep you *really* need, try this little experiment: wait for a time when you're not stressed, such as during a vacation, go to bed each night at the usual time, and see when you wake up naturally, *without* an alarm clock. This gives you a clue as to your *natural* sleep cycle. (Of course, this is assuming you can easily fall asleep and stay asleep—and this may not be the case.)

This book condenses my research on sleep problems into an innovative natural program. It can help you achieve the peaceful sleep you have been looking for through natural approaches to maintaining a healthy lifestyle, relieving stress, and getting a good night's sleep.

Chapter One
Creating a
serene
Sleep Environment

You will probably spend about one-third of your life asleep. Stop for a moment and think about this statement. One-third of your life is for sleep! Are you ready to enjoy it?

Do you have trouble falling asleep? Do you wake up in the middle of the night and find it difficult to go back to sleep? Do you wake up groggy and tired? All of these are signs and symptoms of sleep deprivation and insomnia.

Insomnia is described as difficulty in falling asleep or staying asleep that persists longer than a day or two and interferes with your daytime functioning and quality of life.

Primary insomnia is defined as difficulty sleeping with no specific physical cause. It can be a result of stress, fatigue, anxiety, worry, caffeine, alcohol, or the inability to relax after a fast-paced day.

Secondary insomnia is a symptom of an underlying physical or mental condition that should be corrected or

> Sleep now, O sleep now,
> O you unquiet heart!
> A voice crying "Sleep now"
> Is heard in my heart.
>
> The voice of the winter
> Is heard at the door.
> O sleep, for the winter
> Is crying "Sleep no more."
>
> My kiss will give peace now
> And quiet to your heart—
> Sleep on in peace now,
> O you unquiet heart!
> —James Joyce

addressed by a physician before the insomnia can be relieved.

Your particular sleep difficulties could be a combination of primary and secondary insomnia. But even with underlying medical conditions that are difficult to correct, there are many things you can do to help yourself get a good night's sleep.

Use Your Senses

The first step in getting a better night's sleep is to create a perfect bedroom environment. Sleeping is actually a very sensual experience. When you create the perfect bedroom or sleeping area, remember that all your body's *senses* come into play.

Vision Turn off night lights if they are not needed. Our ancestors relied on the sun to wake them up. Our eyes are very sensitive to even the slightest dot of light, such as that given off by the bedside digital clock. You may be able to get better rest by minimizing available light and turning the clock to face away from you. Some sleep experts suggest sleeping in a pitch-dark

create a perfect

room. Close the shades and curtains. If you don't want to use blackout draperies, try an eye mask to stop visual stimulation. It really works! Several airlines incorporate eye masks into their care packages on long-term flights, so a sleep mask might also help you get some shut-eye when you travel.

Hearing Continuous steady sounds can be soothing and relaxing. However, your body is programmed to note any *changes* in stimulation. Any sudden or irregular sounds may interrupt your sleep cycle and cause you to awaken. (This was a bonus for our ancestors, as the slightest creak, sigh, or whisper could mean sudden death from a wild animal or a marauding enemy.) By contrast, calming, low, and steady sounds like white noise or ocean waves may actually help you sleep. You can buy CDs or electronic gadgets with appropriate, continuous sounds. Some parents find that vacuuming helps their children nod off (and cleans the rug at the same time). If the on/off rhythms of an air conditioner or heater bother you, consider keeping the fan on at all times. Music therapy has also shown benefits, as classical and new age music often aid the brain to begin beneficial sleep-onset activity.

bedroom environment

🍂 *Sensation* Pay attention to temperature and touch. What's the best temperature for sound sleep? Surprisingly, your thermostat should be set to a comfortable 67 degrees in the winter, and 76 in the summer. Adjust and set the thermostat to deliver a comfortable (not hot and not cold) temperature, and then leave it there. Position any air vents away from your face so that you cannot feel the breeze as it is forced through the ducts. Sleep on a good mattress for comfort and sup-

quality sleep comes from *quality pillows*

port. Some people prefer a firm mattress while others like a softer, more cushioned sleep. Use soft, high-thread-count linens that offer breathability. Avoid any polyester clothes or other fabrics that may feel stiff or retain moisture. Wear comfortable cotton instead. Use a cozy down or therapeutic pressure-sensitive foam pillow that does not distort the contour of your spine. I like to use a hypoallergenic goose-down pillow. Down feathers are the fine insulating feathers that are found beneath the larger external feathers of the goose. I do not recommend pillows with these larger feathers, since they may be sharp and poke through the pillow. Quality sleep comes from quality pillows. Down pillows cost quite a bit, but you can fluff them after every use, and they remain like new for a long, long time. They feel light and warm in the winter and cool in the summer. Finally, take a warm bath before bed, smooth lotion on your skin, or try a soothing massage for ultimate relaxation.

Taste Try to go to bed with a clean mouth and teeth. Brush and floss your teeth every evening before bed, and avoid any stimulating foods or drinks thereafter. Skip that last slice of cold pepperoni pizza right before bed. If you do not eat at least three hours before bedtime, the chances of experiencing heartburn and a bad taste in your mouth will decrease.

Smell Keep your bedroom smelling neutral or use a pleasantly scented candle (be certain to blow out the candle before sleep). Your olfactory nerves will enjoy the pleasing aromas. Some people prefer a soothing aromatic powder or spray. Avoid pungent, stimulating scents in the bedroom, such as tobacco, food, paint, or cleaning materials. Remove any potential allergens or any dust or mildew by washing your bedsheets regularly in hot water and vacuuming your carpets. Because of smells and allergies, think twice if your dog or cat wants to sleep with you.

Unclutter Your Bedroom

It's also important to get rid of clutter in your bedroom or sleeping area. This will remove tactile, visual, and even olfactory problems. Organize the visual aspects of your room. Clean up. Straighten your bed linens and clear away the bedside table. Put away things that remind you of daytime problems. Shelve any books that aren't being read. Only have one or two good books or magazines available. I like to keep a notebook next to my bed when I'm in a strong working mode, and I write down all of my thoughts before lying down for sleep. I remove everything from my think tank and put it into the notebook.

You may also suffer from other unnoticed environmental stresses. Some people have problems with electronic devices that produce electromagnetic fields (EMF-producing equipment). In the bedroom, avoid some exposure by placing all electrical equipment, such as alarm clocks, lamps, radios, and television sets, at least three feet away from the bed. Plug in an electric heater to warm you prior to sleep, but don't leave it on all night. Do the same with electric blankets.

Even if you are not sleeping at sea, you will feel better if you make sure that you have "battened down the hatches" and gotten everything shipshape. Make sure that doors and windows are securely locked, that you have a glass of water and tissues at the ready beside the bed, that the

knowing *you*
have done
all you can
to assure
preparedness,
safety, *and*
security
allows for
restful sleep

smoke alarm works, the candles are extinguished, the iron is unplugged, the garbage has been taken out, and so on. It is wise to complete nagging tasks—like finding your income tax return or the light bill or a lost key—before you go to bed so that you won't worry about these problems all night. Or write them down for tomorrow's to-do list.

Many people like to lay out their clothes and paraphernalia for the next day so that there is no stress in trying to find the needed briefcase, the letters to mail, or the socks that match. Put things you need to take with you in front of the door or in the trunk of your car. Knowing you have done all you can to assure preparedness, safety, and security allows for restful sleep.

According to the "Sleep in the City" survey, Detroit, Nashville, Cincinnati, New Orleans, New York, and Las Vegas are designated as cities that can't sleep.

If you live in Minneapolis–St. Paul, Anaheim, San Diego, Raleigh–Durham, and Washington, D.C., you are sleeping nicely.

Chapter Two

undoing Your Stress

Unlike our ancestors, most of us are not suffering from seasonal stress (freezing or starving to death) or sudden-death stress (running from charging bears and wild boars). Most of our stress actually takes place in our mind. It's not outside circumstances that keep us awake at night, but rather what we *think* about. Anxiety-driven stress and peaceful feelings begin in the same place: your thoughts. Even though you feel stress in your physical body, it's your mind that generates this negative tension.

I am originally from Chicago, where the traffic at rush hour can be very anxiety provoking. Recently I was driving to a famous restaurant, anticipating an Italian dinner of Chicken Parmigianino, when I noticed an SUV right behind me, so close, in fact, that I could plainly see the driver in my rearview mirror. He was furrowing his brows, a look of rage on his face because we were moving too slowly. He zipped out of our lane into the one next to us, without signaling, and then rode the bumper of the car in front of him until he could nose in front of me, and then he zigzagged across four lanes with amazing agility, only to be stopped by a red light. When the light turned green, his battle started anew.

> "For fast-acting relief, try slowing down." —Lily Tomlin

As it turned out, we were both going to the same restaurant. In spite of his lane-changing demonstration and fifteen minutes of rage, fury, and hustling, both of us arrived at nearly the same moment. I mention this because I have no doubt that this man has trouble sleeping. He is putting himself under extreme stress because of his inability to control Chicago traffic!

You could be doing the same thing. If you don't learn how to manage stress, it will manage you.

Stress has become such a staple of daily life in America that even children are now experiencing major episodes of stress. The shuffle from school to day care to sports practice and the pressure to do well on homework and

> ## If you don't *learn* how to manage stress, *it* will manage you.

after-school programs has children as stressed as their parents. I should know. My wife and I have a grade-school son and boy-and-girl twins who are always giving us shuffle work. Between guitar lessons, Cub Scouts, soccer games, and schoolwork, my children can become easily stressed unless we make sure that they have fun with what they're doing.

Some stress can be a good thing. Without it, there is no motivation to move—no growth, no change, no accomplishment. If you could live a stress-free life, floating in warm water in a sensory deprivation chamber, you would eventually become stressed from lack of stress!

Think about someone you know, maybe a highly charged individual who, in the middle of great stress and pressure, makes important deals, creates new ideas, and seems to make the world function at lightning speed. This individual enjoys being involved in activities that draw upon his strength and spirit, and give him motivation to do his best. But things begin to break down when there is a shift to *negative stress*. You become detached because you dislike the activity you are involved in. Instead of trying to do your best, you give in to exhaustion and cynicism. Your mind shifts to negative thoughts and you begin to feel tired and ineffective, as if the life were literally being drained out of your body.

These negative thoughts eventually take over even your sleeping hours, and your entire life becomes disrupted.

You can get away from this danger zone by learning how to build an unshakable sense of internal positive power. Your health and your wealth depend on it. Start now to stop negative thinking. Claim your own well-being, no matter what happens around you. If you are having trouble sleeping, don't keep reinforcing this by asking, "Why can't I get to sleep?" Instead, affirm your-self. Make the positive commitment now to get a good night's sleep: "I have had a long, rough day, but now I can sleep and rest. Tomorrow is a new day."

I also practice another method to release stress. I write down all my negative thoughts before going to bed. I have a pad of paper and a pen nearby, and I literally write everything out—I get it out of my head and down on paper. You will be amazed by this technique. It turns bedtime into a time for resting, not thinking, scheming, or worrying. Once you have been able to clear your head, focus on a beautiful and calm image: a person, a work of art, a beach, or anything else that makes you feel good. Close your eyes and focus on the image while taking long, deep breaths. Breathing is very important. Allow your thoughts to merge with your breathing. Feel your lungs expand. Let your muscles relax, starting at your toes and slowly moving up your body. You will probably feel a lightness or tingling sensation. Let the tension dissolve from your legs, stomach, chest, arms, and hands. When you get to your head, stretch your lips and jaw and then relax your facial muscles, your temples, your eyebrows, your forehead and scalp. Think about relaxing every muscle step by step.

claim your own
well-being

Streamline and Simplify

There is also a lot you can do in your home and office to lighten up and de-stress your life. By now, many of us are beginning to realize that more, bigger, and faster are not necessarily better. You are the one who decides how much is enough and what will make you happy. Catch yourself when you notice the hallmarks of burnout coming on. Notice when that negative stress starts to enter your mind and body, and get rid of it immediately. This can become as simple as switching a light on or off. Instead of being a captive of relentless media images proclaiming the need for new cars, clothes, or a fabulous body, take charge of your own mind.

Research in the field of social neuroscience provides insight into this process. Trauma, anxiety, stress, anger, and other negativity create negative activations in the brain stress centers, which can lead to unhealthy and even toxic states. Making the choice to relax and remove negative stress is often the most difficult part of the process. Taking the steps that follow your choice—

supporting your decision—tends to occur with relative ease once a solid choice is made.

Think about the story of a fisherman on the beach. He is busy catching fish, enjoying time with his family, and savoring sun, sea, and sand. But he decides that he should do more. Eventually, after years of effort, he has a whole fleet of employees and fishing boats working for him; he spends every hour in the corporate offices of a large building; he has a cell phone, e-mail, and a company car; and he dreams of the day when he can retire to spend time on the beach, savoring sun, sea, and sand.

Here are some ways to ease the congestion in your life:

Clean up and unclutter your home, car, and office. Feng shui consultants insist that the free flow of the life force through your physical environment will energize you and encourage prosperity, love, and success. Piles of junk in the garage, under the bed, or behind the door will cause energy to "clump" and create negativity. In addition, you won't be able to find things when you need them. Zen practitioners encourage you to store things where they will be most useful: "Hang the bucket next to the well." If you don't have a lot of time for decluttering, just spend fifteen minutes cleaning up what bothers you the most. Perform triage on your stacks of stuff—either use it or lose it.

🖐 *Organize everything* that's left after your streamlining party. Organization experts are available to help you, but you can also do it yourself if you will simply sort through your possessions and keep only the things you like, need, and actually use. Most people have more keys, books, magazines, shoes, kitchen gadgets, tools, and junk than they will ever need. Give away things you don't use and pare down your collections of stuff. Use special organizing shelves, boxes, baskets, and storage units to put things away while still keeping them accessible. It's easier to be serene when you can find everything for your taxes, your law school class, your bird-feeding project, or the Christmas decorations at a moment's notice. You'll find that order is sacred.

🖐 *Manage your time* and schedule your day. Keeping a careful calendar is actually relaxing. You know what you will be doing during the day and you can schedule in important or urgent activities, knowing that necessary actions will be taken and nothing will slip through the cracks. Make use of time-planning books or computer programs or handheld electronic organizers that help to keep you on top of things and remind you of meetings or events coming up. You'll no longer have the stress of forgetting birthdays and anniversaries or missing deadlines. Make time for yourself.

You
are the one
who decides
how much
is enough and
what will make
you happy

Let in fresh air and sunlight.
Modern homes and automobiles are tightly sealed to
be more energy efficient, so you need to remember to
open windows and doors for fresh air and sunshine.
Spend time outside. Replace your plastic plants with
real ones, since plants improve air quality, giving off
fresh oxygen and pulling in airborne pollutants like
carbon dioxide. Ferns are great oxygen producers and
you don't need to have a green thumb to grow them
with success. Get a good vacuum cleaner and use aller-
gy-free cleaning products. Dust furniture regularly and
don't seal yourself in. A stuffy nose may induce night
snoring and disturbed breathing. Run exhaust fans to
get the air moving and consider using a vaporizer to
breathe more freely. Winter furnaces pull moisture
out of the air and desiccate your nasal passages.

Settle for less than perfect. Give it your
all, but don't expect everything to work at 100 percent
of capacity. Accept that people will make mistakes
(including yourself) and won't always be able to meet
deadlines. Offer agreeable solutions when those days
approach. Realize that the sun will still set and the
stars will come out at night whether or not you make
a mistake.

🌂 *Shorten your to-do list.* Keep a notebook or tape recorder handy. If a thought pops up in your mind, write it down or dictate it into the recorder. Then collect these thoughts at the end of the day. Keep a running to-do list with the most urgent items prioritized in some way. Try to get the list down to just three important items every day. Check them off when you're done, and you'll feel a sense of accomplishment. In addition to writing down the three things you *have* to do, add three things you *want* to do. Make sure that you schedule in some fun and relaxation. What are three things you would love to do today? In addition to making a living, you need to remember to make a life.

Cognitive Behavioral Therapy

Cognitive behavioral therapy (CBT) is a treatment approach that focuses on the interaction between mental activity and behavior in the development of disorders. Changing the way we think and act can help in resolving these disorders. We can improve our well-being by learning to cope with our problems in a healthy manner. CBT has been shown to be an effective alternative to drug therapy. CBT works. Studies of over two thousand patients have shown subjective and objective positive effects on sleep.

If you are interested, ask your physician for a referral to a behavioral psychologist who uses CBT. Morin et al. of the University Laval in Quebec, Canada, cites simple and effective CBT methods for relieving insomnia:

❧ *Control stimulus.* Insomnia is associated with arousal and worry, which is then associated with a reinforced context of unsuccessful sleep. CBT emphasizes changing the association to normal sleep.

learn to cope with problems in a *healthy manner*

❧ *Restrict sleep.* Reduce the number of hours you actually spend in bed to only the hours that you have been getting sleep. For example, if you are in bed for eight hours but only get six hours of sleep, you should in fact stay in bed for only six hours, and increase the amount of time as the weeks progress and your sleeping improves.

❧ *Change beliefs and attitudes* about sleep. Faulty thinking gets us into self-destructive modes.

If you are not sleeping, don't worry; lie still, rest, and enjoy peaceful thoughts. Don't dwell on sleeplessness; shift to more positive thoughts. Trying to force yourself to sleep does not make it come more easily.

Learn relaxation techniques. Use relaxation, breathing, meditation, hypnosis, and music therapy to reduce tension and stress.

Music Therapy

What if I told you, "Right now, sing a song?" You would look at me perplexed. But there are studies that show that taking a practical approach to relieving *stress* can have amazing implications on *sleep*. Are you stressed? If so, take a minute, go for a short drive, and sing a song in your car (I sing with my son in the car and we have a great time; we're both Elvis fans) or pick up the guitar and strum a few chords. How about turning on the radio in the living room and performing a nice song-and-dance routine? Right before bed, take a warm shower, and sing some lullabies in the shower. These relaxation techniques work!

You don't believe in the power of music? Well, just look at plants. Green nonthinking creatures respond to music in positive and negative ways. Their growth can improve with the right musical environment. So turn on Beethoven and get an earful tonight. Play whatever music makes you relax. Music is inexpensive and non-addictive, has no side effects, and will work every time.

Medical Hypnosis

Hypnosis or hypnotherapy can sometimes be used to initiate a positive immune response, intervene in pain control, and even help with chronic medical conditions such as anxiety disorders. The word *hypnosis* originates from the Greek word for *sleep*. Freeman et al. of the Michigan Hypnosis Institute found that people who were taught self-hypnosis were able to strengthen their immune system through increasing their IgA, an immunoglobulin marker. In addition, medical hypnosis was also helpful in dealing with conditions like skin problems, irritable bowel syndrome (IBS), and nausea and vomiting. If you are a smoker, medical hypnosis could help you in dealing with acute stress and in breaking the smoking habit.

Hypnotic pain control is a great technique because it helps you isolate your pain from the rest of your healthy body. It also allows you to imagine or visualize the pain. Anyone who can't sleep because of arthritis or chronic pain may benefit from working with a medical expert trained in medical hypnosis.

Techniques for Stress Relief

"Stop. Look. Listen." You've heard this before, and it's usually from a parent telling a child to take a moment to *think*. It's simple to slow down—just stop, look, listen. Rest and feel at ease once again. Employers can let employees have a moment to slow down and rest during the daytime. As an employee, remind yourself to set limits to your workday. Zombies aren't needed at work. Top performers get a balance of exercise, time at work, and a great deal of rest. Ask them when they go to bed, and you may be surprised that they will tell you at 8 or 9 p.m. Some people aren't in bed until midnight each night, but they get a solid night of sleep. So you don't need to compare your pattern to that of others—you just need balance.

Slow down. Your work will be there for you in the morning. Delegate your responsibilities as much as possible. Everyone tells me that they need to do more of this. Things that others can do for your will save your work hours and help you coordinate a complicated day. Most people feel proud when asked by another for their expertise and help in accomplishing a goal.

Take a look at your work surroundings. Are they comfortable? Or do they add stress to your day? Take away any clutter, or hire an assistant for one day a week to help you organize. Write down your daily plans, don't carry them in your head. Leave the work *at work*. My wife is a human resources executive for a major bank corporation. She's wonderful at her job. I'm the extreme opposite. That is, I'm good at my job, but I tend to favor working much longer hours that reflect my medical training. In fact, I built a full kitchen and a shower in my office just to make my work environment comfortable. I'm often there for twenty hours at a time. But in the real world, the eight-hour day should be sufficient to finish your work. I believe in a well-designed office environment. Keep it comfortable and use your senses. Is it too loud? How comfortable is your chair? Is your computer at the right angle and height? If not, you may unnecessarily suffer at night from lower back pain, neck pain, or similar annoyances. If you work in an environment that has heavy machinery, dirt, or other chemical or environmental hazards, make sure to take off all your work clothes at your front door, take a nice shower, and then slip into some comfortable lounging clothes for the evening. This practice is sanitary and will help you in your transition toward a good night's sleep. Remember how Mr. Rogers always changed his shoes and jacket when he came home? These are good, practical habits to incorporate immediately.

Some useful and simple stress-reduction techniques:

Limit your exposure to stressful situations. Take frequent breaks,
rest periods, and vacations whenever possible.

Learn to say no to any additional projects.

Meditate, do yoga, or go in for a therapeutic massage.
Take care of your mind and your body.

Stop and take several deep, calming breaths. Deep breathing
calms and relaxes your body by supplying increased oxygen to your
bloodstream, which decreases fatigue and anxiety.

Avoid alcohol and cigarettes. Substitute these habits with more
healthy alternatives such as physical exercise,
talking to friends, and healthy eating.

Chapter Three
Improving Daytime
performance

Overcoming Jet Lag
and Shift Work

Hectic lives and erratic work schedules play havoc with the healthy sleep patterns of millions of people.

🍂 *A best-selling mystery author* dreads finishing her latest book. Why? Her publisher intends to send her on a tour of seventeen cities as soon as her book is in print. She pictures herself chatting with fans, signing autographed copies in bookstores—and lying awake in a strange hotel every night as she jumps from time zone to time zone.

🍂 *A dedicated straight-A student* pulls a couple of all-nighters getting ready for a big exam—and then discovers he can't sleep when he gets the chance.

🍂 *An intensive-care nurse* is thinking of switching jobs. She loves her work, but every week she pulls a twelve-hour shift that upsets her sleep schedule and makes it impossible for her to relax when she's not working.

🍂 *A newly retired couple* expects to enjoy world travel after they collect their pensions. Instead, they find that the speed of supersonic jets plunks them down in strange cities before they can adjust. "I keep looking at my watch to see if it's bedtime yet," the husband says. "And if it is, then what? I can't go to sleep on cue."

We love speed, movement, and getting things done. Many of us do shift work, as more businesses have decided to stay open 24-7. Radio announcers, doctors, and factory workers are just some of the millions faced with demanding schedules. How can we wind down from the stresses of our day? Is there anything we can do to restore our fractured sleep patterns?

First, you should, as much as possible, think of your work shift as being *consistent*. Request from your employer that your shift be as consistent as possible; let them know that you will perform better with a reasonably consistent schedule. Do your best to stay with your sleep-wake schedule even on your days off, including weekends. If you work at night and sleep in the daytime, maintain this balance even when you don't have work scheduled. Make your bedroom dark. Close the shades and sleep (even if it is daytime out), set your sleep times, and make sure others know your boundaries. At work, make certain you have adequate light, as this will activate your brain into thinking

> Half of all Americans who work report that sleepiness on the job interferes with the amount of work they get done.

it is daytime, even if it's dark outside. This is the science of chronobiology working in your favor.

You should also avoid antihistamines and other narcotic hypnotics. Many shift workers develop dependencies on drugs, alcohol, and stimulants. If you currently drink to get to bed, you are actually causing your body to dehydrate. You will likely feel relaxed prior to bed, but alcohol can alter your dreams, your breathing, and possibly your heart rate, and will increase the amount of work on your liver and kidneys. Dehydration will make you thirst for more water, and you will likely wake up during the night for a drink, thus interrupting your sleep.

> Sleep deprivation costs employers an estimated $100 billion in lost productivity, sick leave, medical expenses, and property damage.

Antihistamines inhibit the histamine sites in your cells and make you drowsy. If taken on a long-term basis, antihistamines can actually cause changes to your immune system.

My natural sleep solution offers you long-term help. Natural options will reset your sleep-wake cycle for a consistent night's sleep without the side effects. Don't look to short-term solutions of a quick fix; you need to establish a life strategy for sleep, natural sleep, the way you slept as a child.

Dietary supplements are a great choice for people stuck on a daily antihistamine or other drug, who may be looking for an out but know they need some supplemented help to initiate or maintain sleep.

Natural Sleep Aids

A solution for both shift work and jet lag can be found in taking some of the natural sleep aids that provide a mild sedative effect for relaxation and improved quality of sleep. For example, melatonin is a hormone naturally produced by the pineal gland in response to light and darkness, reaching its peak production at night. Melatonin helps to establish normal circadian circles of sleep and wakefulness. As we age, the pineal gland can become calcified and release less of this hormone, which also appears to regulate a system of self-repair and regeneration for the body's tissues as well as promoting restful sleep. Melatonin is not a narcotic but rather an antioxidant that fights free-radical damage and helps many people achieve calming deep sleep. It is often suggested for insomnia, nervousness, anxiety, and restoring normal sleep patterns in response to jet lag. According to evidence from several randomized, placebo-controlled trials, individuals who took melatonin the evening after arriving at their destination point and continued to take it for a few days after arrival were able to establish a normal sleep pattern. Even more, individuals were able to improve their sleep latency period (the amount of time it takes to initiate sleep) while also increasing their level of daytime alertness. By helping initiate sleep even a few minutes earlier then normal, melatonin will decrease irritability and help with establishing a healthy sleep-onset time.

establish a
life strategy for sleep

People who suffer from delayed sleep-phase syndrome have a problem with sleep latency, and melatonin can really help. Consider taking 0.5 to 3 mg of melatonin an hour or two before going to bed. I also recommend 0.5 to 3 mg of melatonin for anyone who has insomnia. This is a very small dosage and is recommended so that you don't develop a tolerance to melatonin or receptor insensitivity. Try this first before moving on to standard pharmaceutical therapy like benzodiazepines or other sleep aids.

In addition to the benefits for sleep initiation, melatonin is considered a great supplement to preventing problems associated with oxidative damage. Antioxidants are an important part of your life. By floating through your system, they keep a close guard on the free radicals (oxygen atoms that have a negative charge and can cause damage to your cells and DNA). The antioxidants bind to these free radicals, and your body is able to delete these now neutralized molecules from your system. Melatonin also offers health benefits for dealing with attention-deficit disorder, bipolar disorder sleep problems, high blood pressure, and cancer.

Valerian root is another natural sleep aid, an herb that has a relaxing effect on the nervous system and helps you feel fresh and rested in the morning. It has been used for centuries to promote relaxation and restful sleep. Studies show it can decrease the amount of time it usually takes to fall asleep. It is not addictive. Valerian root extract may not have an immediate effect on all people; multiple doses over a two-week period may be needed to see significant improvement.

Adverse effects for valerian are rare and minor, such as headaches or dizziness. Alcohol should be avoided, even though there is no evidence of "potentiation" (an increase of valerian's effects if you ingest alcohol). Based on reviewed studies, the most effective dosage for valerian root extract is between 200 mg and 600 mg. This is a safe and effective herbal choice for insomnia, and can also help as a calming agent for daytime stress, aggression, and anxiety.

Both melatonin and valerian root will most likely be safer and healthier than drugs prescribed for sleep. Hypnotic drugs can become addictive and have additive effects with other narcotics or medicines. Drugs can also cause serious side effects and rebound effects (worsening insomnia if you abruptly discontinue the use of the drug). Problems like amnesia (memory problems or loss of memory), tolerance (the drug loses its effectiveness if used repeatedly with time), cramps, vomiting, shaking, and sweating are other side effects that have been associated with drugs for sleep. The worst problem is dependence. You may become addicted to these sleep drugs, and withdrawal symptoms may be severe. Natural sleep supplements like melatonin and valerian root can help wean you off these drugs.

The Consequences of Poor Sleep

Getting a bad night's sleep can lead to disaster, as it's difficult to make clear decisions when you are tired. According to the National Sleep Foundation's 2005 "Sleep in America" poll, 60 percent of adult drivers (over 160 million people) said that they had driven a vehicle within the past twelve months while feeling drowsy. Over 100 million people admitted to actually falling asleep at the wheel! Take a moment and think about the

Getting a
bad night's sleep
can lead to
disaster, as it's
difficult to make
clear decisions
when you
are tired

harm you could do to yourself and to others. Opening
your window, taking in a breath of cool air, chewing a
stick of gum, or drinking caffeine-
filled sodas won't help you keep
alert. The only way to stay alert is
to get a good night's sleep. Make
the decision now to never drive
when you are tired. To emphasize
this point, the National Highway
Traffic Safety Administration conservatively estimates
that over 100,000 *police-reported* crashes are the direct
result of driver fatigue each year. This leads to over 1,500
deaths, 71,000 injuries, and $12.5 billion in monetary
losses. Larger-scale accidents are often the result of
poor sleep as well: both the Chernobyl disaster and the
Exxon Valdez oil spill were directly attributable to
sleep deprivation.

> Drowsy driving causes
> over 100,000 car crashes a year!

Chapter Four

relaxing the
Body, Mind, and Soul

On a recent business trip, I was feeling extremely stressed and just couldn't get to sleep. I decided to try a new approach. I requested a therapeutic massage from a licensed professional and was amazed at the relaxation I felt. I almost melted into the sheets, peacefully drifting off to sleep without a care in the world.

Therapeutic massage is a wonderful sleep aid. It can help with sleep disorders that have a neuromuscular origin, such as pain, tension, involuntary muscle contractions, and restless leg syndrome. Research shows that when a daily massage is given for a period of ten days, even adults with chronic fatigue syndrome feel better. Massage therapy turns off the sympathetic nervous system (fight or flight) and turns on the parasympathetic system (rest and digest). If you can't afford to be treated by a professional, your mate might be willing to engage in mutual back rubs. A good back massage can reduce nerve irritation and increase the production of pain-killing endorphins. Some people find vibrating electrical massage gadgets helpful—but any relaxing touch can soothe knotted muscles and relieve stress. We all have the need for human touch. "Mate massage" can help a couple reconnect. Try giving your mate a short nightly massage before sleep. Many

> "Tension is who you think you should be. Relaxation is who you are."
> —Chinese proverb

people also find that spa visits, combining water, steam, and massage, help them to relieve stress.

Sleep difficulties are often made worse by short-term or low-grade pain. How can you sleep when something hurts? Pain usually feels worse at night because you're no longer involved in the busy daytime world. There you are, in bed, in the dark, alone with a headache or backache. No wonder you can't sleep. One very effective pain reliever is a combination of hot/cold therapy and therapeutic massage. A hot bath or a cold pack can relieve pain, and massage helps with muscle aches. Massage can ease a backache. Don't sleep on your stomach, as this arched position can hurt your cervical spine at the neck level. Sleep on your side with a straight spine, or on your back. Those with a snoring problem should choose a side position, since back sleeping encourages snoring. You'll need an adjustable pillow that supports your head and neck. Don't hang on to a lumpy or thin pillow. Getting the right pillow will help you sleep and protect your spine.

> Go to bed earlier in gradual steps, fifteen minutes earlier each week

Relieving Hospital Insomnia

Sleeplessness is a common problem for hospitalized or bedridden patients. Consequently, there has been a search for nondrug alternatives for the treatment of insomnia. Massage has been found to be an effective alternative option. A study conducted at the University of Arkansas concluded that back massage is very useful for promoting sleep in older men, even those suffering from a critical illness.

Soothing Your Child

My wife and I have three children, each one so loving and different from the others. When our son was an

Therapeutic massage
is a wonderful sleep aid

infant, he was an angel. My wife and I said that we created him as a gift for all the difficulties in our lives; he was a source of great calm. When our twins came around five years later, all hell broke loose. Most parents can relate to this. The boy twin would wake up in intervals the exact opposite of the girl twin. They were extremely restless, so I started lightly massaging their backs, feet, hands, arms, and legs. The substance of the massage is the light touch and soothing action between two people. Comfort is shared by both child *and* parent.

Even fretful babies and restless children sleep more peacefully after a massage. In one study of children and adolescents, those who received a thirty-minute massage each day for five days in a row slept longer and more soundly than those who had no massage at all. In addition to helping an infant or child sleep, the calming touch of a parent establishes a valuable opportunity to soothe and nurture your baby. Research shows that as little as fifteen minutes of massage a day significantly benefits infant weight gain and mental and motor development.

Techniques of Therapeutic Massage

Swedish massage is a smooth, flowing style that
improves relaxation, circulation, and range of movement.
It also relieves muscular tension.

Deep-tissue (neuromuscular) massage is intended to
reach the connective tissues, tendons, ligaments, and nerves.
It helps to release tension areas called "trigger points."

Sports massage focuses on specific muscles, tendons,
and ligaments that affect athletic performance and
that may have been injured during activity.

Reflexology massages specific reflex zones on your feet
to relieve tension and pain. Many believe it can also
improve circulation in areas of your body
corresponding to these reflex zones in your feet.

Chapter Five

eating right
for Better Sleep

One natural way to improve sleep is to eat a nutritious diet and keep your weight within a normal range. Doing so can relieve a host of sleep problems, including night eating, sleep apnea, and heartburn or acid reflux. Some studies show that if you don't get enough sleep at night, you may be prone to overeating in order to keep going during the day. It's a dangerous cycle—you don't get enough sleep, so you eat more to make up for it, and then you gain weight and suffer disturbed sleep, and you become fatigued during the day, so you eat more, and so on.

A study conducted with the University of Wisconsin medical school found that individuals who sleep less than eight hours a night have a higher body mass index (BMI) than those who sleep eight hours or more a night. BMI is a measurement of fat in the body. A BMI over 25 indicates that you are overweight. Results from the test indicated that individuals who slept less had lower levels of leptin, a hormone that regulates appetite. A researcher at the University of Chicago has found that when people lack sleep, their body displays changes in leptin and grhelin. They have higher levels of grhelin, which activates hunger, and lower levels of leptin.

> Approximate Ideal Weight (in pounds)
> Male: 106 + (height in inches over 60 x 6)
> Female: 100 + (height in inches over 60 x 5)

Mood swings can also cause you to change your eating habits. Take care not to lose your temper or have arguments before bed. Some people even suggest that, in order to get to sleep quickly and easily, you avoid watching the news at night.

Night Eating

Night eaters can be at serious risk for a number of health problems. Sleep should be a time when your body rests from digesting food and works on maintenance and repair. Walking around in the middle of night and foraging for food is not healthy, especially if you are already overweight. Nutritious, balanced eating and vitamin supplements are the escape route from night-eater syndrome. People who get most of their calories in the middle of the night are likely to be very overweight.

Eating a high-protein dinner with a little fat may help to reduce hunger pangs at night. But don't eat too close to bedtime, as protein helps to maintain alertness. Make sure you drink a lot of water during the day so that your body is properly hydrated. Thirst can often be mistaken for hunger. It is best not to drink a lot of water right before sleep because you may have to take restroom trips during the night, which contributes to broken sleep patterns.

Sleep Apnea

Sleep apnea is characterized by disruptive snoring and gasping for breath during sleep. It is made worse by excess weight. Many people are not even aware that sleep apnea is the reason why they awaken every morning feeling very fatigued. Their sleep partner may also suffer from similar distress.

Some doctors don't consider sleep apnea to be a true sleep disorder, but rather a disorder of respiratory-related physiology that interferes with restful sleep. Nevertheless, estimates are that at least one out of every two hundred people suffers from it, and most don't even know they have it. Today in sleep centers, overnight monitoring and polysomnography are used to diagnose the condition. "Apnea" refers to episodes of shallow breathing where at least 50 percent of the airflow is reduced. Estimates are that among middle-aged adults (age 30–60), as many as 24 percent of men and 9 percent of women suffer from this problem, which results in daytime sleepiness, impaired concentration, and fatigue. But because you are asleep during all of the nighttime choking and gasping, you may not even know you are

> Howard Taft, 27th president of the United States, often fell asleep while signing important documents and speaking with members of Congress. He most likely suffered from obstructive sleep apnea.

doing it. Sufferers can have apneic episodes from thirty to a hundred times a night, yet studies suggest that only one out of eighteen people with sleep apnea are properly diagnosed, and only 50 percent visit their doctors about this sleep difficulty.

Increasing age (over age 35), being male, and being overweight are all risk factors for extreme snoring and sleep apnea. Obstructive sleep apnea (OSA) occurs when the airflow ceases as a result of a temporary blockage of the upper respiratory airway. Most experts believe this occurs when there is a sleep-induced failure of the throat muscles to hold the airway open and the suction created by efforts to breathe. The period usually lasts ten to ninety seconds and is terminated by a brief arousal (waking up from sleep and then falling asleep again). Long-standing sleep apnea and excessive snoring are often associated with higher blood pressure and even risk of diabetes and heart disease. An apparatus called a Continuous Positive Airway Pressure (CPAP) machine consists of an air pump and a mask that can be

Do you have recurrent headaches? Do you snore? Then you should check with a sleep specialist. You may have a sleep disorder such as sleep apnea or hypoxemia. You probably aren't getting enough oxygen to your brain, thus the headaches. In addition, your body probably has a high level of carbon dioxide.

worn over the mouth or nose at night to keep air passages open. The CPAP apparatus works. As uncomfortable as it may be in the beginning, you will learn to adjust to wearing one, and you will be more alert in the daytime.

Not all snoring is related to sleep apnea. If you snore and sleep on your back, try sleeping on your side or stomach instead. You can even wear a device at night that reminds you not to roll over on your back. Pneumology research in Brussels, Belgium, recommends position training to overcome sleep apnea. You can sew a pocket in the back of your pajama shirt and then place a golf ball or tennis ball in the pocket to force you to sleep on your side instead of your back.

Heartburn and Indigestion

What you eat and drink can definitely contribute to sleep deficit. If you are overweight and older, you need to take extra care in this area. A cup of tea can have enough caffeine to keep you awake all night. This is because as you age, deep sleep becomes more fragile and your body becomes more sensitive to stimulants.

Don't eat a heavy meal within four hours of going to bed. A large meal causes an insulin spike, and insulin helps the body to store fat. Stay away from pickles, MSG, spices, and any foods that give you indigestion, gas, or heartburn. Acid reflux occurs when the flow of stomach acid backs up into the lower esophagus—not a pleasant sensation, and likely to disturb sleep.

Food to Dream About

A recent article by Yana Golbin, a sleep specialist in Chicago, is very helpful in addressing the connection between a healthy diet and healthy sleep.

Which comes first, poor sleep or poor diet?

Which comes first, poor sleep or poor diet? Is fatigue due to diet, or are we just too tired to cook well-balanced meals and take the time to eat them? In our society, food is perceived as an enemy. Does our society of "super-size combos" and "just-add-water meals" affect our sleep? Most specialists say "yes," with such added causes as alcohol, caffeine, and bad eating patterns. It has been proven that a poor diet negatively affects energy, ultimately causing what is commonly known as fatigue.

Negative pressure on the physical being can put stress on an individual and alter sleep patterns. Caffeine, especially consumed in the evening in the form of coffee, caffeinated tea, chocolate, soda drinks, and certain pain relievers increases the heart rate, which may lead to restlessness and an inability to fall asleep. In addition, caffeine before bedtime may also lead to nightmares, dehydration, and morning fatigue.

Over-eating, or what researchers call "midnight-eating," may also lead to poor sleep. Eating light, small portions of food and sticking to the basics of the USDA's Food Guide Pyramid provides nutrition for the body to regenerate during sleep, eases digestion, and hydrates the body for morning and next day energy.

It is especially important to eat breakfast. The body processes energy in the form of complex carbohydrates, providing longer-term energy in its raw form; just the opposite of its counterpart of simple carbohydrates, which provide bursts of energy, leading to unstable highs and lows. The best time to consume carbohydrates is at breakfast.

Eating late can cause more than poor sleep. A researcher at a Chicago Veterans Affairs Hospital has shown that eating and then lying down within two hours can cause Gastroensophageal Reflux Disease (GERD). GERD is characterized by the stomach acid leaking back up into the esophagus due to a weakened sphincter at the top of the stomach. The sphincter weakens during food intake. The intense acidity of the stomach matter causes a sensation of what is generally called "heartburn." If you need to eat before bedtime, make it a light snack at least two hours before sleep.

The optimal diet has been shown to begin in the morning with a larger-than-usual breakfast consisting of breads (cereal, bagel, etc.) and fruit; lunch may include a sandwich, soup, or salad; and dinner may consist of small portions of protein, fruits, and vegetables. Eating every five hours gives your body time to digest the food and convert it to energy. Also remember that some foods interfere with medications, such as cranberry juice, herbal tea, and some spices.

Sleep Is for Warriors

He who sleeps best wins—at least that's the evidence that years of sleep studies are beginning to show. Studies indicate that after eighteen or more hours without sleep, your reaction time will slow down from a quarter to a half second or longer. So what does this mean for a jetlagged, world-traveling athlete, hoping for peak performance in the next day's match? Or for a student hoping to score an A on an exam after pulling an all-nighter? Delays in reaction times will likely keep you from success.

A deep restful sleep (and plenty of it) is the foundation of a better golf score, tennis match, Olympic run, and maximum productivity at the office. But because people are leading busy and stressful lives, they are stressed and are not getting enough sleep, and therefore they cannot achieve their ultimate success. If the ancient Roman gladiators and the contenders in Olympic games routinely slept ten to twelve hours a night to prepare themselves, who are we to store up a major sleep debt—sometimes for years? Whether we are professional athletes, sports lovers, or just people who prefer chart-topping success at the office—we need our sleep! Sleep deprivation leads to increased accidents, health problems, poorer sports performance, and lower academic and work performance.

Doctors, kinesiologists, and health-care professionals usually endorse a steady routine (a daily exercise program and activity) and advocate going to bed at the same time—*every night*—as sleep-promoting therapy. If you want to perform at your best, you should know that your body moves naturally through a period of rest, sleep, and alertness called the sleep-wake cycle. The body regulates sleep by the time of day, in cycles known as *circadian rhythms*. The term "circadian" means a rhythm with a period of twenty-four hours. This rhythm is fundamental to our human body clock.

What's important is the *kind* of sleep you're getting. Insufficient dreamtime in REM (Rapid Eye Movement) sleep can result in irritability, anxiety, depression, interrupted concentration, and decreased ability to handle the complexities of modern life. The health consequences of sleep deprivation also increase the potential for abuses such as using too much alcohol, smoking, or taking drugs, stimulants, narcotics, and other sedatives to balance the disrupted sleep-wake cycles.

Plato, a fourth-century BC Greek philosopher, insisted that "bodily exercise, when compulsory, does no harm to the body." But don't overdo it. Plato was said to have died in his sleep at the age of eighty following the festive wedding of one of his students. Perhaps due to too much Greek dancing!

Human Growth Hormone and Sleep

The human growth hormone (hGH) is secreted by the pituitary gland in the brain and helps regulate many of the body's muscular activities, improves physical

A deep, restful sleep
(and plenty of it)
is the foundation of
a *better* golf score,
tennis match,
Olympic run, and
maximum
productivity
at the office

strength, and reduces fatigue.

In a study of fifty men and women over age 67, half of the individuals did forty-five minutes of aerobic exercise three times a week, and the other half did only stretching exercises three times a week. At the end of the six-month study, those from the aerobic group were able to spend 33 percent more of their sleep time in deep sleep than they did prior to the study. The aerobic exercisers also increased their production of hGH, which is released only during the circadian cycle of sleep. Those who only stretched without much exertion saw little improvement in deep sleep, and did not show increased hGH production.

The time of day one exercises also seems to impact sleep. In Finland, researchers studied 1,600 people between the ages of 36 and 50, and found that exercising later in the day (between 4 p.m. and 7 p.m.) seemed to play a role in developing a deeper sleep state. The possibility of increased body temperature could have offered some additional sleep support. A hot or warm bath at night produces this similar passive heating at bedtime and can also help induce sleep.

Exercise has been shown to decrease the time it takes to fall asleep and to develop REM sleep. However, those who really push themselves physically, such as body builders, long-distance runners, and gymnasts, need longer restful sleep sessions to build muscle and rebuild stretched and damaged muscles.

Antioxidants for Better Sleep

During the daytime, your body utilizes your nutrition as you go about your daily activities. But what happens at night, when you need to rebuild and recharge? Your body turns to its reserves. At the end of the day, your physical reserves of nutrients and antioxidants, which support your immune system and fight free-radical damage, are at their lowest level. Before going to bed, take a multivitamin as well as a powerful antioxidant. These will help replenish your reserves for the evening repair session.

Most people have a fatty meal for dinner that contains minimal antioxidants. You really should be eating oranges, strawberries, blueberries, and other natural antioxidants during the evening hours, when antioxidant levels in the body are at their lowest. Make a fresh fruit smoothie or take a dietary supplement. Antioxidants taken an hour or so before sleep time are important for those who suffer from sleep apnea or other problems that limit the oxygenation of cells in the body.

Some healthful sleep solutions:

Exercise on a regular basis, but avoid overexertion.

Build a routine for sleep.
Just like working out, create the habit of going to
bed at a particular time each night.

Think of the 5 senses to help you sleep better:

SIGHT—turn off all lights.
SOUND—reduce sounds, or play relaxing, soothing music
in the background.
TASTE—practice proper oral hygiene before bed, by brushing and
flossing your teeth. Avoid eating late at night, and allow for
at least two hours before bed after finishing your dinner meal.
TOUCH—use soft clean pillowcases and blankets as well
as a firm comfortable bed.
SMELL—use clean sheets and spray soft scents on your bedding
for a sense of calm.

Take proper nutrition supplements, which can help prepare for
a more relaxed state of mind prior to sleep, and they contain helpful
antioxidants to rebuild and recharge a healthy body and immune system.

Reduce sources of "stimulants" (tobacco, coffee, and caffeinated drinks)
during the day, and avoid them a couple of hours before sleep.

Try these steps to get a better night's sleep and
you will definitely have a happier, more productive day!

Chapter Six

Using *gender-specific* Techniques for Sleep

Sleep problems vary for men and women.

For Women

Women can solve the PMS dilemma naturally. A better wording for PMS is *temporary hormone imbalance*, which can encompass perimenopausal, menopausal, and postmenopausal women. Menopause is a natural process of the body. Related sleep problems are very common among women, and this is the reason most drug advertising for sleep aids is directed toward women. According to the North American Menopause Society, nearly forty million women in the United States are past the age of spontaneous menopause—age 51 and older. Some 40 percent of menopausal women may suffer from sleep problems, including hot flashes, restless legs, sleep anxiety, night sweats, excessive stress, and other frustrations. That's more than sixteen million American women who rarely get a good night's sleep!

> "Of scenes of nature, fields and mountains;
> Of skies, so beauteous after a storm—and at night the moon so unearthly bright,
> Shining sweetly, shining down . . . I dream, I dream, I dream."
> —Walt Whitman

Even though menopause is a natural chronobiologic process, deep, restful sleep may be disturbed in many menopausal women for a number of reasons. Studies show that better sleep leads to better health and better daytime functioning. Gaining more control of the sleep function could help women in menopause enormously, restoring a feeling of calm, control, and peaceful relaxation during an often difficult time period. And it's not just women over 51 who suffer. The transition right before menopause, perimenopause, which occurs even before menses have ended, may also be a stressful and frustrating time for women where sleep is concerned. Productive daytime functioning may be disturbed if a woman doesn't get enough relaxing sleep, and this leads to more stress, anxiety, and frustration—a debilitating cycle. Some women are almost afraid to go to bed because they know they'll toss and turn, or wake up in the middle of the night and worry because they aren't sleeping.

gaining more control of the *sleep function* could help women in menopause enormously

Before taking synthetic hormones for PMS, first consider a few natural options such as supplements, bedtime tea, life changes, and relaxation techniques. Foods considered high in *estrogenic compounds* will help with the natural supplementation of the hormones your body is missing. Soy, apples, cherries, potatoes, and wheat-based foods are examples of what you can increase in your diet. Sleep supplements such as melatonin and valerian root help with relaxation.

In 1991, the NIH prepared clinical studies evaluating the usefulness of hormone replacement therapy (synthetic drugs) on menopausal women. In 2002, the study was canceled due to the development of increased risk of ovarian and breast cancer. Heart disease, blood clots, and strokes were also noted. The natural way is the safe and effective way.

Vitamins

By combining particular vitamins and bioflavonoids (natural chemicals from fruit having bioactive benefits on the body), you can also achieve a sense of balance and at least a reduction in the symptoms of menopause.

Vitamin B complex

Vitamins may help alleviate many of the problematic symptoms of menopause. I first recommend vitamin B complex. B vitamins are water soluble, so they will not be stored in your body's fat cells. If you have low levels of vitamin B, you will likely be cranky, irritable, fatigued, and depressed. Therefore, eat those leafy green vegetables and nuts, beans, and fish. Consider at least 25–50 mg of vitamins B3 and B6, and 200–300 mcg of vitamin B12. Folate is necessary for neurological development in pregnancy at 400 mcg per day (180 mcg per day for an adult female who is not pregnant). Because folate lowers the level of homocystine (which can cause heart problems and osteoporosis), make sure to take vitamin B6 and B12 along with the folate supplement. Folate can also help with depressive symptoms.

Vitamin C
Vitamin C is nature's healing vitamin, beneficial for cell growth and immune function. For women especially, vitamin C can help prevent the oxidation of LDL cholesterol, which is great for heart health. Vitamin C also assists your metabolic functioning. It can help with vascular capillary strength and integrity of blood vessels.

Vitamin E
This is considered the "menopause vitamin." Vitamin E may relieve hot flashes and also help in the psychological symptoms of menopause. Green leafy vegetables and eggs are high in vitamin E. However, a dietary supple-

ment is probably your best form to achieve a benefit. I recommend at least 20 IU of vitamin E.

Flavonoids

Flavonoids are found in many fruits and can help boost the immune system. They also protect against free-radical damage of the cells. I recommend grapes, prunes, berries, and pomegranates for premium flavonoids, ones that will help your immune system and keep you healthy. For women, proanthocyanidins (a type of flavonoid) from berries are a must; these are the phytochemicals responsible for keeping pathogenic bacteria away from the cells of the urinary tract and other parts of the body. If you are prone to urinary tract infections, take at least 36 mg of proanthocyanidins from rich blue and red berries (not from pine bark extract). Blueberries and cranberries are the best. These are also great for women who have problems with menopausal vaginal problems and menstrual bleeding.

Soy

Soy is good for alleviating hot flashes and maintaining healthy cholesterol levels. Just drinking soy milk or eating tofu can help, or supplement with a high-quality dietary supplement. Although the scientific literature on this is mixed, soy can help decrease the number of hot flashes and migraines associated with menopause. As a

**A few quick solutions to lower
the number and intensity of hot flashes:**

Maintain a healthy diet and eat the right foods
(plenty of natural fruits and vegetables).

Limit alcohol consumption.

Stop smoking.

Decrease coffee drinking.
Caffeinated drinks can elevate blood pressure and
increase the risk of hot flashes. Instead, replace with a
bedtime tea (chamomile) and cold drinks to cool the body.

Exercise regularly (some hot flashes can be eliminated by
exercising and doing yoga).

Wear comfortable, breathable cotton underwear and clothing.

Take vitamins and minerals.

Drink water regularly.

supplement, doses between 50 and 75 mg per day of soy isoflavones are helpful. If you consume a soy protein drink (not isolated isoflavones), then you will likely need 30 to 50 grams to have an effect to get the dosage of isoflavones. This can also help with maintaining good cholesterol levels.

For Men

Over time, the male body tends to experience a decrease in testosterone levels. This can lead to a lack of energy and a decrease of the sexual drive.

Exercise can improve blood flow. Men with erectile dysfunction can improve their physical abilities over time by exercising the pelvic floor muscles. You can feel these muscles at work if you try to stop the flow of urine when you're using the bathroom. To exercise these muscles, sit comfortably and "flex" them ten to fifteen times in a row. Don't tighten your back or stomach muscles at the same time, and don't hold your breath. Exercise can also help with body weight and therefore decrease your problems during sleep. As you gain weight, the laryngeal area also increases in size, and you may develop apnea problems. Work hard at losing that extra ten pounds and you will likely see a great difference in your daytime performance and nighttime rest.

Sleep deprivation is now at an epidemic level, and this has an impact on relationships and health. Sleep apnea in men is very common, along with snoring. Using a CPAP apparatus (a small mask attached to an air compressor, which forces air into the lungs) will help with breathing. This is a simple solution to sleep apnea and should be diagnosed by a sleep medicine physician. You will find that when you use this device, your daytime alertness will increase, you will have more energy, and you will likely lose weight as a result of the increased activity.

Men should avoid consuming alcohol up to *two hours before bedtime*

Research from the University of Wisconsin shows that men have a 25 percent increase in sleep-related breathing disorders after consuming alcohol. Men should avoid consuming alcohol up to two hours before bedtime. Women with minimal to moderate alcohol consumption do not have an increased risk of developing sleep-related breathing disorders.

Chapter Seven
Caring For
children,
the elderly,
and
special needs

Children

Watching a child sleep brings peace, comfort, and joy to anyone, and if you are blessed with twins or multiples, you get double the joy!

With children who have problems sleeping, guidelines are needed for both the parents *and* the children. Pre-sleep practices, maintaining good sleep throughout the night, and waking up refreshed and alert are going to be your focus when helping a child sleep.

> "Those who claim to sleep like a baby do not have one."
> —A parent

An infant or baby may not be able to tell the difference between day and night. With an infant, life is a bit difficult until about five months of age, when the sleep cycles begin to foster.

Sleep deprivation in a child can lead to excessive daytime sleepiness, hyperactivity, and, ultimately, behavioral and academic problems at school. This is why it is very important to set schedules for sleeping and waking up.

With children, the key is routine and ritual. Keep this in mind for any sleep help. Make certain the sleeping environment is fit for a king or queen. Remember, our *first* approach is to correct the sleep environment. It should be cozy, clean, and organized, and should establish the correct senses (temperature, feeling, etc.).

For an infant, wrap the baby comfortably and play rhythmic soothing music or rock and sing to the baby. Lightly massage the body, especially the hands and feet, and rub the baby's back prior to falling asleep. Make this a ritual prior to bedtime. For a crying infant, you will likely learn to discriminate between crying due to hunger, upset or pain, or need for a diaper change. Wait and react to those cries that require full attention; otherwise, allow the infant a chance to adjust for a few minutes. Comforting a baby is also good but can lead to a dependency on this ritual. Let the baby make noises and movements, as this is part of the sleep cycle adjustment. Try to delay your responses to get up and check on the baby.

Minimize your infant's anxiety as much as possible. At less than a year old, babies should be spoiled; hug them as much as possible, and if you leave the baby for the evening with a babysitter, make sure the babysitter and the baby bond for a while before the baby is put to bed. Breast-feeding mothers should be careful of what foods upset a baby. Minimize any foods that have caffeine or other stimulants that may be passed to the baby. Also, certain foods may cause gas in a child and increase the colicky response. When your child is no longer breast feeding, remember to add only one food each time to make sure you know what is affecting the baby.

Teething babies often have difficulty sleeping.

Offering a cold teething ring or frozen food prior to sleep will allow your child to reduce the amount of pain in his or her mouth. Keep an eye on any child with food in his or her mouth, and do not place food or bottles in his or her bed, as this is a choking hazard. Just hold the child while he or she gnaws on a frozen cookie.

If your child cries excessively during sleep, he or she may be suffering from sleep apnea or other breathing-related issues, such as nasal obstruction. Consult a physician and discuss this. In the meantime, you may want to hold the child and gently touch them until they are calm and the crying episode has finished.

> "Adam and Eve had many advantages, but the principal one was that they escaped teething." —Mark Twain

When traveling with a baby on an airplane, make sure you are equipped with the proper bottles for a child when the plane takes off and lands. Sucking a bottle will prevent or at least limit the baby's ears from popping and will reduce irritability. For an older child, provide some food or a stick of gum for chewing at takeoff and landing.

As your baby grows to be a young child, continue giving him or her the right foods at the right times. Avoid fatty foods at night, or at least two hours before bedtime. The best advice is to give your child a snack of vegetables or fruit in the afternoon and then a healthy family dinner.

Have your child take chewable vitamins about an hour before bed. Stay away from sugary vitamins before sleep, as these can cause dental cavities. All children, beginning as soon as the teeth start to come in, should practice good dental hygiene. Have your child brush his or her teeth with you before going to bed. Make this a ritual. I recommend an electric toothbrush, which stimulates the gums and the child. Have fun brushing!

A child from one to three years old may want to be comforted for bedtime. Some parents sleep with their

continue giving them the ***right foods*** *at the* ***right times***

child. This is a personal decision, but it does offer reasurance. By limiting the child to his or her own bed environment, you will establish boundaries. Just maintain the reassurance of the child to build self-confidence and to help him or her overcome fears of darkness, thunder, and those dreaded monsters.

Remember to exercise the little rascals! Have your child get good activity after school. Many schools have recently dropped their physical education programs altogether, and with the surfeit of enticing computers and video games, children need to be encouraged to spend time in active outdoors play. Have your child run laps around the backyard, take out the trash, help with washing the car, and do fun activities to engage in movement. Our son plays soccer and basketball. He loves interacting with his friends, and on these days he comes home ready for sleep. Exercise is great for the heart, muscles, coordination, friendships, leadership and teamwork skills, and to help with sleep.

Establish set sleep times and wake-up times. Announce, "It's eight o'clock, time to go to sleep." Then help your children brush their teeth, do a prayer, and tuck them into bed or lead them to the bedroom. Make sure your child uses the restroom prior to going to bed. If your child has a problem with bedwetting (enuresis), restrict the amount of fluids prior to bed and use urination-alarm techniques such as the SleepDoc, which gently vibrates and causes the child to change sleeping position.

Night terrors usually occur during a deep stage of sleep. The child screams in confusion and terror. After a few minutes, he or she usually falls back to sleep or wakes up without remembering what has happened. These are not considered nightmares and may continue into adulthood. Let your physician know if your child experiences these more than once a month. They may lead to changes in EEG (brain measurements) and EKG (heart measurements) when the person becomes an adult. Although it may be a natural episode, night terrors should be looked at by a physician for potential injury and to identify causative reasons. Make sure your child doesn't get hurt in these episodes. Try to calm your child down through reassurance and use a cool, moist towel to wash his or her face, as this may help calm down or even end the episode.

Nightmares are normal dream states that offer drama to a daytime event or association. They usually happen in the last third of sleep and are not the same as night terrors, which usually happen in the first third of sleep (deep sleep) and are much more dramatic. Children usually recall what a nightmare was about. This is not the case in night terrors. Just comfort a child by explaining that nightmares are normal parts of dreaming—some dreams are nice and others are nightmares.

Sleepwalking (somnambulism) may cause injury to a

Bruxism, or teeth grinding,
is a common problem seen in some children.
When the teeth grind at night, the surface layer of teeth is lost.
This can lead to serious dental problems. See a dentist as soon as you are aware that you or your loved one have bruxism. The dentist can fit a simple mouth guard to avoid teeth destruction.

child. Restrict the sleep environment if there is a risk of danger. Safety is the main concern. Keep the child on the main or bottom floor so he or she doesn't run the risk of falling down stairs. Check the type of medications that the child is on, as this may be a cause of sleepwalking. Don't irritate a sleepwalking child because he or she can become strong and violent. These individuals usually have amnesia about the event (they cannot remember anything). As a side note, most episodes in *adults* happen after a preexisting stimulus interrupts their sleep, and medications, illicit drugs, and alcohol can also cause sleepwalking. For sleeptalking (somniloquy), change the child's position or rub his or her face with a warm, moist towel.

In the morning, wake up consistently at the same time, even on weekends. Have the child make his or her bed so that the organization of the room is preserved. Since some children (and parents) prefer having the clothes ready for the next day, select them the night before. In our family, we have a "Monday through Sunday" clothes dolly that is hanging in the closet with the entire week of clothes ready for our son. He selects the shirts and pants for the week, and there are underwear and socks ready in each hamper as well.

Set a nightly ritual like prayer by the bed. Children will learn to enjoy the emotional benefits and reduce any anxiety prior to sleep. When a child appears anxious and unwilling to sleep, chose a soft-yet-firm approach to comfort or assure the child. Usually this is an issue from ages 3 to 7. A calm friendly talk at night will help the child fall asleep peacefully and may help with parent-child bonding. I sit next to our child and talk to him quietly prior to bed about the good things in the world, how soft the pillows and sheets are, and how comfortable it is to be there. He usually falls asleep within a couple of minutes to the sound of my "radio voice." I close my "radio talk show" with good night and sweet dreams in Greek: "*Kali nihta, kai oneera glika.*" My mother used to reassure me and my brothers this same way. Don't rush this sweet moment. Take a few minutes to relax yourself and enjoy your child's presence.

> "The only thing worth stealing is a kiss from a sleeping child."
> —Joe Houldswort

With adolescents, maintain similar sleep-wake timing. Offer adolescents advice on controlling the hours that they must be in bed for sleep. Let them know that this is the time they are going to have another growth spurt in their lives, and they need their sleep to rebuild their bodies and look their best. I would also recommend to them that if they sleep well, their immune system will be prime, and they will be more productive and less tired in the daytime. Regular sleep can often help adolescents decrease their acne symptoms. Also, many hormones are regulated in the sleeping period, and a regular sleep schedule will help with controlling irritability.

The Elderly

Older people typically exhibit poor sleep efficiency. A melatonin supplement will help to accelerate the onset of sleep. Anyone over the age of 50 should benefit from a 0.5 to 3 mg dose of melatonin.

as with anything,
talk with your physician
about starting any new plan

Thirty percent of people over age 50 suffer insomnia, which results in other associated problems. Consider that if you have difficulty falling asleep, and then wake up several times during the night, and then have problems falling back to sleep, this will take its toll on your body. In addition, older people tend to wake up earlier in the morning. These changes cause increased daytime sleepiness and problems with attention and memory, and also affect the mood of the individual. This can be corrected with a dose of melatonin thirty minutes or more before sleep (up to two hours prior to bedtime). Of course, as with anything, talk with your physician about starting any new plan. If you consider the physical, neurological, and other health benefits of melatonin and getting a good night's rest, I think you will be pleased with the response. A study done at the Massachusetts Institute of Technology demonstrated that patients who were provided even physiological doses of melatonin (0.3 mg) benefited by significantly improving sleep efficiency.

By helping increase total sleep time, you can also relieve daytime fatigue. The more activity an elderly person has, the better health that will result.

Special Needs

Kids and adults with special needs will greatly benefit from a good night's sleep. Many neurological disorders may lead to problems with attention, and may be a result or cause of sleep deprivation. Oftentimes sleep problems are associated with medications taken for neurological disorders.

Many people with special needs are hypersensitive. Therefore, make sure all the lights are dimmed prior to bedtime. Turn off the television and muffle any other

**A few possibilities for parents of children
with special needs:**

Try to reduce stress.
Work on reducing any jealousy among siblings, and let them know
not to be embarrassed around peers. Most people recognize your situation,
and if they don't, they need to learn.

Learn and teach patience.
Don't become frustrated. Take a moment and regroup.

Recognize stresses beforehand and try to deal with them
before things get too hectic. For example, if you know it takes time
to dress, allow enough time in advance of an event to do so.
No big deal if you are late.

Ask questions.

annoying sounds that may be in the area. Remember, the
sleep environment is an important part of getting
good sleep.

Speak with your physician about adding a sleep supplement for the nighttime period if the individual is

taking stimulant medications in the daytime. Adding sources of amino acid–rich foods (especially those that contain theanine and tryptophan, which is converted to melatonin by the brain) will help a person relax. For example, a nice cup of yogurt, herbal tea, an egg, or some nuts eaten at night may help tremendously.

Individuals with intellectual disabilities can suffer with sleep problems. In addition, their parents oftentimes also have associated sleep problems likely due to stress. Because many of these individuals have repetitive behaviors or compulsions, it is important to understand the needed physiologic and behavioral response to help people gain the sleep they need.

Chapter Eight
Understanding
pets
and Sleep

〜

Americans own an estimated sixty-five million dogs and an astounding eighty million cats, and we spend over $7 billion each year on pet food, pet toys, and pet care. Owning pets is a good investment because they have a calming effect on adults and children.

However, sleeping arrangements can be a source of conflict—for both the pets and their owners. Pets are wonderful additions to a family, but when the bedroom environment is disrupted, people can have serious problems, and so can their pets. My recommendation is to consider the bedroom space as sacred ground and teach your pets not to sleep in your bed. Remember, the first area we pay attention to with sleep is the sleep environment. Engage in activities with your pet during the daytime and relax with it in the evening, but leave your room to yourself when it's time for sleep.

Pamper Your Pet

Pet owners know the passionate bond between a dog or cat and their daily lives. Often pets are treated as equal members of the family. Pets are great therapy for cancer patients, people with hypertension, and disabled individuals. They offer companionship and an actual reduction in high blood pressure. However, we also know that the biorhythm of pets begins to synchronize with those of their human owners over time. This presents problems for sleep-wake cycles. For example, if your dog wakes up frequently during the evening, you will also experience some of these activities. Heart rates and breathing frequencies may also alter as a result of this cohabitation.

The solution: make sure certain boundaries are set. If your pet is determined to sleep in your bed, it's time to purchase a comfortable bed for the pet. You can position the "pet bed" next to your bed. The emphasis is on removing your pet from being your sleeping companion. In time, and with proper direction, your pet will understand, and you will both enjoy pleasant nights of rest.

If **your pet** is determined to sleep in your bed, it's time to *purchase a comfortable bed for the pet*

In Japan, therapy centers have begun to commercialize the health benefits of animals by incorporating animal petting locations to help people reduce stress. This appears to be an effective tool in cities where animals are not allowed or in busy cities such as New York, where having pets may be more difficult or not allowed by condo associations.

A study from the University of Missouri at Columbia demonstrated that walking a dog five times a week helped subjects lose an average of fourteen pounds over a year. What motivation!

Beyond the pet's benefits to your sleep and health, did you know that sleep apnea can also happen in animals? If you recognize that your pet is having problems, don't forget to mention this to your veterinarian the next time you are in the office. Disorders like narcolepsy, bed-wetting, and nightmares are found in animals as well. Dogs sleep an average of ten to thirteen hours a day. When animals have illnesses, they sleep more than normal, just like we humans. Therefore, any time your pet is sleeping more than usual, it may be an indication of a health problem.

Chapter Nine
Using
natural
Supplements
and Nutrition

The demand for sleep aids has increased to the point that private companies are now investing current research and development dollars to provide health professionals and patients with safe, healthy sleep aids and dietary supplements with therapeutic effects. The United States Government and the National Institutes of Health, as well as major university medical schools such as those at Harvard and Cornell, have applied millions of dollars and countless hours of research to understanding the health benefits of natural supplements and alternative medicines.

As a medical doctor interested in cutting-edge research, I have turned my attention to the power of plants to provide therapeutic benefits, using botanical sources such as vegetables, fruits, and herbs containing natural phytochemicals, and applying this to health benefits.

Many of today's medical and health-care professionals lack adequate training and information in understanding the significance of complementary and alternative medicine (CAM) in treating sleep disturbances. After reviewing the literature for natural medicines, it is clear to me that both anecdotal and clinical studies report several CAM advantages, ranging from effectiveness in relieving symptoms to lowered financial cost. In addition to herbs and natural remedies, many alternative-therapy techniques such as acupressure, massage, aromatherapy, meditation, relaxation therapy, and yoga may assist in subjective feelings of well-being and aid in better sleep.

As CAM becomes an important component of allopathic medical training, meeting exacting standards in natural medicine and therapeutic delivery systems will be of great interest for product development, safety, and efficacy.

Extracts from a number of botanicals, including valerian root, chamomile flower, passionflower, and hops have been shown to be useful sleep aids. Lavender (a hypnotic aromatic agent) has been reported to improve quality of sleep. Certain minerals, vitamins such as pyridoxine HCL, amino acids such as taurine, and melatonin have all been used as natural therapeutics to regulate body rhythms and alleviate insomnia.

Many of these herbs, vitamins, minerals, and other natural alternatives have been approved by the Food and Drug Administration as GRAS (Generally Recognized As Safe). But others need additional research and clinical studies.

Currently, several different raw-materials suppliers in a variety of locations provide minimum requirements for their products. The marketers of natural products must seek to use standardized components in their formulations. Development of common standards for all suppliers will be important to the future of CAM.

Safety and Side Effects

Some studies show possible harmful interactions between natural sleep aids and other medications or herbal remedies. Some patients taking natural alternative medicines have reported problematic symptoms

Consumers, physicians, and health care providers need to be *aware of foods or other natural alternatives* that may interfere with sleep

that may conflict with proper sleep. For example, hawthorn, widely used in Europe in the treatment of congestive heart failure, has been associated with tachycardia, headache, dizziness, abdominal discomfort, sweating, fatigue, agitation, and sleeplessness.

Consumers, physicians, and health care providers need to be aware of foods or other natural alternatives that may interfere with sleep. Caffeine, for instance, has a direct effect on sleep/alertness states. Many need their cup of java to get started in the morning and complain of sleeplessness when they drink coffee too late at night. Many products other than coffee also contain caffeine.

I feel that three of the most helpful natural substances to support restful sleep are melatonin, valerian root, and L-theanine. I add antioxidants to the sleep time to help prevent breakdown and rebuild the body and wake up refreshed.

Melatonin—the Third-Eye Sleep Hormone

Your sleeping ability may be connected to what many people have called your "third eye," the little-known pineal gland. Even though many of us have trouble sleeping, this tiny gland creates and releases nature's most restful sleeping potion. It's called melatonin.

Located at a point corresponding to the location of the "third eye," behind the forehead, the pineal gland is able to convert the "feel good" hormone, serotonin, into melatonin—under the influence of light changes. Melatonin is stored for release from the pineal gland during periods when light is dim or scarce.

Ideally, the pineal gland increases the supply of melatonin while you are asleep during the night and then shuts down production as day dawns. The gland responds gradually to changes of light in the environment, waking you up or putting you to sleep.

Melatonin is superior to many sedatives because although it induces sleep, it does not affect critical REM sleep, or "dream sleep," which is so important to a restful night.

People who travel extensively often use products containing melatonin to help them maintain a normal schedule even after crossing several time zones—allowing them to overcome jet lag and get restful sleep even though normal circadian rhythms have been disrupted.

Clinical studies with melatonin involving children and adults have been promising for both those with normal sleep patterns and for those with insomnia. Particular benefits (i.e., sedation) are found in patients with low melatonin levels. Melatonin supplementation is very effective in elderly individuals even though melatonin levels do not necessarily decline with age and individuals with normal levels can still report insomnia.

Research studies have indicated an effective initial dosage is 0.1 up to 1.5 mg daily, consumed two hours or less prior to bedtime, and then a gradual increase in the dosage until an effective level is attained. However, high melatonin doses (over 1.0 g) may cause side effects and disrupt the mechanism of the circadian system. Current research from the Massachusetts Institute of Technology recommends as little as 0.3 mg for an effect.

Data on the safety and efficacy of melatonin as a supplement are still limited. Currently, there have been reports of depression, hormonal alterations, renal insufficiency, fatigue, and cardiovascular side effects. Melatonin should not be taken by patients who are breastfeeding or pregnant, or by those on warfarin.

In summary, melatonin appears to be effective, safe, and well tolerated in the treatment of those patients of all ages suffering from insomnia, from circadian abnormalities, and from jet lag. Melatonin may also be a safe alternative to traditional hypnotics.

Valerian Root

Valerian root is another promising natural sleep aid. It is an herb that has a relaxing effect on the nervous system and leaves you feeling fresh and rested in the morning. It has been used for centuries to promote relaxation and restful sleep. Studies show it can decrease the amount of time it usually takes to fall asleep. In dietary supplements, it is standardized to an exact dose of valerenic acid. It is not addictive.

Products that contain both melatonin and valerian root as well as a combination of other ingredients can reduce the side effects of too much caffeine and promote relaxation, decrease stress, and improve the quality of sleep.

L-Theanine

I'll call L-theanine the "Relaxation Amino Acid." This amino acid is very similar to L-tryptophan, but I don't really recommend L-tryptophan. The reason is that there is considerable medical and laboratory evidence behind L-theanine that far exceeds the benefits of tryptophan. If you are trying to cope with debilitating stress and anxiety (who isn't?), then try L-theanine before going to a mood-altering medication. Unless you want to welcome side effects of drugs, this is a must-try. In addition, this amino acid improves concentration and lowers the jitters seen in coffee drinkers.

So what is L-theanine? It is an amino acid found in tea. Why do you think tea drinkers are able to have their caffeinated tea and not have the jitters that you see in coffee drinkers? Research shows that L-theanine helps the body relax by quickly being absorbed through the small intestine and going directly to the brain to generate what are called alpha waves—awake yet relaxed frequencies for our brains. It may also play a role in the formation of GABA, a neurotransmitter that is important for relaxation, sleep, and memory. You should look for products containing 50 mg of L-theanine and up to 200 mg. It should also contain pure L-theanine (avoid any mixture of D and L, as they may be inferior and not as efficacious).

L-theanine can reduce stress, promote relaxation,

improve the quality of your sleep, and improve your work and learning performance. It can also help women who have PMS symptoms and reduce the negative effects of caffeine. Get ready to relax and turn your mood around.

Hopefully dietary supplements such as these, not requiring a prescription, will become a first choice for stressed people on the go.

Antioxidants for Sleep

I'm proud to state that I am the first to promote antioxidants during sleep. I have to make this statement because I believe in the benefits of antioxidants and their ability to ward off disease. Furthermore, I'm very big on berries. Blend them if you can . . . raspberries, blueberries, any that are blue or red in color. Bears and animals that hibernate for long months love berries. You should too. These fruits have special phytochemicals called phenolics.

Phenolics have antioxidant benefits and can prevent dangerous oxygen free radicals from causing damage to your cells. Now, what if you drink juice in the morning, have your fruit and wonderful daytime antioxidants, but then as you near the evening, you switch to meats, starchy potatoes, and nutrient-depleted foods? This is considered the normal diet for Americans and the growing diet for the world. By evening, most individuals lack the antioxidants in their bloodstream to protect themselves against cellular damage caused by stress, smoking, overwork, and other harmful agents.

Bears and animals that *hibernate* for long months love berries

This is precisely why you need to take antioxidants at night. Sleep is a time of recovery. Help armor your body with the antioxidants it needs right before going to bed. Most antioxidants will last and offer protection for about eight hours in the bloodstream before being eliminated by the urinary or hepatic system. I've added a potent proanthocyanidin ingredient to my daily regimen. Proanthocyanidins offer antibacterial benefits and antioxidant benefits. The particular proanthocyanidins from certain berries (like blueberries) can ward off your next cold, bacteria trying to lodge onto your respiratory system, or bacteria fighting to grab onto the cell walls of your urinary tract system. In the morning, you will be more energetic and less groggy then ever before.

The government has a great program that can be used by everyone. Take a moment to look at the "Body and

Soul, Colors of Health" and the "5-A-Day" programs. I know these will have a huge impact on our growing youth and many people who want to take a look at what fresh foods should look like and how they help us. Each day add one additional fruit and vegetable to your diet until you feel great. There's green (beans, peppers, spinach), yellow-orange (corn, carrots, tangerines), red (pomegranates, strawberries, watermelon, tomatoes), blue-purple (berries, plums), and white (mushrooms, garlic). If you incorporate a healthy diet, you will reduce your risk of heart disease and even cancer. In August of 2003, the National Cancer Institute worked with the FDA and formed a wonderful health claim:

Diets rich in fruits and vegetables may reduce the risk of some types of cancer and other chronic diseases.

Read that a few times; it's really a part of how we should live. Take a simple step right now and have a plum, an apple, or an orange. Feel the goodness and live life. Tonight that little fruit will be working for *you*. That's powerful. Now you have some armor for the night and for waking up refreshed.

Vitamins and Minerals Can Improve Sleep

Taking proper vitamins and minerals may prevent trouble falling or staying asleep. Too much copper, especially if taken prior to bedtime, may increase the occurrence of nightmares by overstimulating the creative areas of the brain. Foods such as grapes and chocolate contain high levels of copper. As a result, cutting back on these foods prior to sleep may help.

Calcium, on the other hand, can help alleviate restlessness. A glass of warm milk at bedtime may help with relieving muscle cramps. For those who are lactose intolerant, taking a daily vitamin that offers a therapeutic dose of calcium may be a good choice.

A magnesium deficiency can detract from getting a full deep sleep. Symptoms may include waking up at the slightest noise and sleeping additional hours during the day. Diabetics are especially prone to magnesium deficiency. They can acquire the magnesium they need through natural sources, including nuts, broccoli, spinach, and fish.

Every cell in the body needs the B vitamins (B1, thiamine; B2, riboflavin; B3, niacin; B5, pantothenic acid; B6, pyridoxine; B7, biotin; B12, cobalamine; and folic acid), particularly nerve cells. This is best exemplified by folate deficiency, the most common nutritional deficiency in the world. Women who are pregnant must have folate to avoid neural tube defects in their offspring. Vitamin B deficiency manifests itself in neurologic disorders, and thus in sleep problems and muscle weakness. Vitamins B12 or B6 can also help in the therapeutic plan for depression.

P. Chan et al. investigated the safety and efficacy of vitamin B complex capsules in a double-blinded, placebo-controlled study in elderly patients with severe nocturnal leg cramps. After three months of the study, 86 percent of the patients taking vitamin B had prominent remission of leg cramps, whereas the placebo group experienced no difference. The frequency, intensity, and duration of nocturnal leg cramps were reduced. Vitamin B complex is a relatively safe and effective alternative that clinicians should consider in the treatment for nocturnal leg cramps.

Chapter Ten
Developing the New
you

Your longevity, your physical appearance, your good health, and your productivity can all be threatened by poor sleep habits. Sleepwalking through life like a zombie is a high price to pay for trying to have it all, do it all, and be it all. Sometimes the best sleep management program is simply getting your affairs in order, taking charge of your own life, managing your time for optimum health and well-being, and getting organized once and for all. In other words, you might be able to reduce your sleep problems if you learn to incorporate structure and routine into your life.

> Instead of allowing life to rush you along, you can:
> 1. Make time for sleep.
> 2. Learn to use new gadgets.
> 3. Cultivate learned competence.
> 4. Reset your body clock.

Make Time for Sleep

Research shows that most of us need around eight hours of sleep a night to operate optimally, so in your daily planning, be sure to set aside enough time for some solid rest.

Deep down, perhaps you feel that not taking time to sleep is a sign that you have a meaningful, busy, fun-filled life. You are a person of status and power and the world can't do without you while you take time to sleep. Your wagon is so full that you cannot pull it. Year after year, in keeping with our workaholic culture, many busy Americans skimp on sleep, rev up on coffee during the week, and try to catch up on weekends. Then, they may sometimes sleep as much as ten or twelve hours at a stretch. In 2006, according to many surveys, as many as 70 percent of Americans said they got fewer than eight hours of sleep during the work week. Yet most experts agree that we do need a consistent eight hours of sleep to function properly, although there are exceptions.

You can't really catch up on weekends. The reason? Getting fewer than seven hours of sleep a night can upset your body's natural circadian rhythms. Your body goes through several cycles of light sleep and deep sleep each night, and you need around eight hours to get enough of each cycle.

"Somnorexia" is a new word used to describe the sleep habits of busy people who purposely deny themselves sleep in order to squeeze more things into their day. Just as anorexics deny themselves food, somnorexics deny themselves needed sleep. If you're sleeping ten hours a night on weekends and much less during the week, loading up on coffee to stay awake, you could be wreaking havoc in your life. Many otherwise healthy people notice a drastic decline in memory and mood when they don't get enough sleep, but they press on anyway. Somnorexics

"Somnorexia" is a new word used to describe the **sleep habits** of busy people who *purposely deny themselves sleep* in order to squeeze more things into their day never get enough sleep on a regular basis. They skimp on sleep for weeks at a time and finally crash.

Learn to Use New Gadgets

Perhaps you don't sleep well because you fear you won't get up in good time. Begin by getting a good alarm clock—one that wakes you gently or playfully or happily—not jolting you awake with gunfire or screeches or nasty buzzes. Why add to your stress? You can buy an "animal sounds" alarm clock, or one that wakes you with pleasant sounds from nature, such as soft rainfall or ocean waves. There's even a Zen alarm clock said to produce a bell-like tinkle as you slowly wake up. (The chime sounds at shorter and shorter intervals, helping you to slowly emerge from your dreams.) You can purchase "progression wake-up" clocks, which give you your favorite sounds of rainstorms, mountain streams, songbirds, or ocean surf at gently increasing volume level until you're finally awake. All are pleasantly timed to nudge you gently awake.

For maximum sleeping pleasure, get a clock with a snooze button. A snooze button allows you to tap the clock and drift off for a few more minutes of bliss. If you're pressing it too many times, however, the sleep you're getting is fragmented, not restful. Maybe you need an earlier bedtime!

For a more natural wake-up, try a clock with gradually increasing light intensity. (This kind of gradual wakeing up is also useful for the hearing impaired.) Some wake-up clocks allow your light to begin thirty minutes before wake-up time, glow with increasing intensity, and wake you up without making a sound—just like the sun.

And don't forget aroma. You can add scented capsules to a compartment on the top of some light clocks where they'll be heated by the warmth of the bulb, release their scent, and delight your sleeping nose as you awaken.

Studies show that babies are not the only ones who benefit from having a definite bedtime and listening to soothing music to lull them to sleep. Many find that music distracts and relaxes them, calming them before bed. You can get a CD player with an automatic turnoff. Some alarm clocks also have a sleep function that plays music but turns the sound off automatically after twenty minutes or so.

Cultivate Learned Competence

Psychologists have long known that negative feelings inhibit sleep. "Learned helplessness," a phrase used by psychologist Martin Seligman to describe the defeated, passive behavior of laboratory dogs submitted to electric shocks they couldn't escape, is a reaction many of us may feel when we see ourselves as helpless, passive victims trapped in our busy lives. So why couldn't a deliberate effort to gain control and build up our competence in small ways have the opposite effect?

You don't have to believe everything you think. You can monitor your passing thoughts and deliberately choose those that make you feel more empowered and less stressed. You can also learn to be more stress-resilient by living in the moment—taking more time to enjoy relaxed meals, going for a leisurely stroll after dinner, enjoying a sunset, stopping to smell the roses.

action is the antidote to *worrying*

Attitude is everything. During stressful situations, you can stay relentlessly positive, tell yourself that things are going to work out and that you will handle whatever life decides to send you. After all, you've made it this far, haven't you? You can learn to respond in more effective ways instead of giving in to panic. You can slow down, breathe through it, and keep your feet moving.

Action is the antidote to worrying. Learn to take some

small but effective action instead of fantasizing and avoiding. Mail the letter. Clean out one drawer. Make the phone call. Write and mail the check. Answer the e-mail. Fix the squeaky hinge. Change the lightbulb. Donate unused items to the shelter. Baby steps will get you there and, over time, can have a cumulative impact that makes your life more serene. Any sort of action reduces anxiety. Doing is the opposite of worrying.

One simple remedy for both stress and depression is spending time outdoors in the natural world with sunlight and the beauty of nature. Gardening and walking may be relaxing and stress-relieving forms of activity. Limiting use of caffeine may help, along with some form of professional counseling or therapy to fight the worrying "monkey mind" that jumps from problem to problem all night. The mind loves to solve problems, but you can't do much to change things while lying in bed. Put your focus elsewhere. Recall some of the wonderful times you've had as a family. Focus on what you are grateful for in your life, and you'll lighten your mood. It's hard to be grateful and irritated at the same time.

Reset Your Body Clock

Centuries of responding to the regular daily cycle of light and darkness have created humans that respond naturally and automatically to the rise and fall of light. These rhythms govern your digestion, energy regulation, sleep and wake times, and hormone levels. They're like an internal body clock, and are greatly affected by light of any kind. This includes electric light and computer screens. Photosensitivity to light is strongest at dawn. And if too much light is around, as is the case with electric lights, the body may not register that it's getting to be time for bed.

Rhythmic fluctuations of body temperature are consistent and predictable. For example, your metabolism wakes up with the sun and heats up when you eat breakfast. Body temperature reaches its apex when the sun is highest in the sky—between noon and 2 p.m. Then in the afternoon, there's a drop. This is possibly the best time for a nap. In America, we refuse to take a siesta and drink coffee to keep going. By 9 or 10 p.m. or so, for most people, body temperature begins falling in preparation for sleep. At night, when you sleep, body temperature drops naturally. Night owls feel the drop later, around midnight.

The human body is programmed by the biological clock to experience two natural periods of sleepiness during the 24-hour day, regardless of the amount of sleep we've had in the last 24 hours. The primary period is between midnight and 7 a.m. and the second (less intense) period is in the afternoon after lunch. Circadian rhythms are affected by the amount of light you get during the day. Even exposing yourself to an hour a day of bright outdoor light can help to keep your internal clock on schedule, so if you can, try eating lunch outside or taking a walk outdoors. Use sunscreen and know that sunlight can elevate your mood, give you energy, and shift your body clock to an earlier cycle. At night, avoid bright overhead lights. Lamps are more calming. If you wake up too early in the morning, try to get by without turning on a lot of lights. Calm your nerves. Exercise every day, but complete your workout at least a few hours before bedtime. Exercise heats things up. Since eating a meal means food needs to be digested and burned, a major meal just before bed makes things hotter, not cooler. Some people do like a bedtime snack, especially one containing milk.

Think in New Patterns

A recent study conducted on over 23,000 Greek adults supports the idea that napping could reduce the risk of heart attacks. In fact, the study is one of the largest ever conducted on the health

> Sleep well. Be healthy.

effects of napping and shows that a half-hour nap three times a week lowers your risk of dying from a heart attack by a whopping 37 percent. Whether these results prove to be conclusive or not, it is a compelling argument to give it a try. Take advantage of a short nap at work and you will be recharged for the day and a better work performer—making the right decisions and feeling good about your outcomes. The Mediterranean daytime siesta and eating habits may have a strong influence on health. Take note and make some simple changes in your life. Think about lowering your cardiovascular risk factors, such as blood pressure and low-density lipoproteins, as well as cholesterol levels. Take a nice nap, don't smoke (or limit the quantity and timing), get regular exercise, and keep your weight down. These all help with sleep.

A recent study in the *Journal of the American Geriatrics Society* reported that individuals who napped between 2:00 p.m. and 4:00 p.m. did better on mental ability tests—both on the day *of* the nap and the day *after* the nap. In addition, as long as you nap between these time periods, it should not affect your evening sleep.

Balance is what we are missing. It's no wonder that, although we are the richest country in the world, we are not the healthiest of the industrialized nations. Other nations outlive us, and perhaps sleep better as well. Most of us—not all—are warm, safe, and well-fed, yet we do not allow ourselves the time to actually enjoy life. We just try to race through it.

It may be helpful for us to take another look at the way we think and the way we live. This section is titled "Think in New Patterns," but actually I encourage thinking in *old* patterns—those that kept my Greek ancestors healthy and happy in Crete, and the same healthy life patterns that

Mediterranean daytime siestas and eating habits may have a *strong influence on health*

flourish in the lands along the Mediterranean sea: Greece, Spain, Italy, France, Morocco, and Lebanon.

"Think Greek" is one way to look at it. The Greeks were long proponents of moderation in all things—the "Golden Mean." People envied for their longevity, such as those on the island of Crete, most often live in multi-generational families, sit down to a home-prepared meal of fresh unprocessed foods each evening as a family, and are known to sleep, get up, and perform daily routines on the same set schedule most of their lives. They exercise in meaningful activity outdoors, stay close to nature, and enjoy life's seasons in simple natural ways. Perhaps if we followed their example, we could learn how to make our own lives fuller, richer, and a little more peaceful—always conducive to proper sleep.

Nicholas Dunkas, M.D., of Northwestern University in Chicago, published a wonderful book entitled *The Works of Hippocrates*. In this classic reading of Greek history, Dr. Dunkas emphasizes that Hippocrates laid the foundations of scientific medicine as we know it today. The art of medicine included practical applications of the physical world (fire, earth, water, and air) and equilibrium. Sleep was a part of the development of health and lack of it was seen as a cause of disease. He was aware of this in the fifth century BC. Bravo, Hippocrates!

Strive for a Contented Life

Perhaps a contented life is the true magic secret to perfect sleep. A contented life requires a number of components. Eating well, living well, and sleeping well are all part of a much-needed lifestyle change. Human connections, love, affection, family, and community are critical for happiness and contentment. Long-term isolation in our cubicles or apartments is bad for us. The more contact and healthy interactions we have with friends, colleagues, and family, the more likely it is that we can sleep happily. There is more to work than competition and getting ahead of everyone else. Team spirit and cooperative, collaborative efforts reduce stress and turnover, and improve job satisfaction. Liking your co-workers and having good friends at work keeps you happier on the job. And feeling productive at work certainly can make you more content.

> "Sleep that knits up the ravell'd sleave of care, The death of each day's life, sore labour's bath, Balm of hurt minds, great nature's second course, Chief nourisher in life's feast."
> —William Shakespeare

Your mind needs physical exercise as well as your body. You can nurture mind, body, and spirit by getting enough fresh air and exercise, avoiding chemical, physical, and emotional stressors, using supplements or nutrients when needed to optimize functioning, and managing your health, integrating all the activities of daily life into a harmonious whole.

Relax and Receive

You can eat faster, work faster, dance faster—but you really can't sleep faster. Sleep takes just as long as it does.

Do what it takes to reduce stress and give yourself a

peaceful, serene environment to live in. Do you really know how to relax?

Going with the flow, staying fully present in the moment, meditating, learning to relax, getting centered and balanced, and living in gratitude are all ways to help you relax and receive.

If you feel that life is abundant and there are many good things to do and enjoy, you will find yourself better able to relax and enjoy these good things. Would you play a symphony twice as fast to get to the end sooner? Of course not. Sleep also requires its own good time to be refreshing and rejuvenating.

It all starts with oxygen. If you are keyed up and anxiety ridden, you may find yourself short of breath and breathing shallowly. You can practice simple breathing exercises to help yourself relax, like breathing in through your nose, counting to three, and breathing out through your mouth. Start monitoring your breath to calm your-

sleep requires its own good time to be *refreshing* and *rejuvenating*

self. Start thinking positively. Enjoy the realization that you are safe and life is abundant and purposeful. Learn to embrace change.

Yoga is a surprisingly effective alternative treatment. Some yoga classes are devoted to combating insomnia with breathing, meditation, chanting, and basic poses (asanas). Yoga treats the underlying issues that keep people up at night. There is good evidence that people who have trouble sleeping are chronically anxious and aroused. Insomnia sufferers tend to have higher-than-average levels of adrenaline and cortisol (the stress hormone) pouring through their bodies. Yoga coaxes down these hormones. Practicing yoga at any time of day reduces cortisol by bedtime. If you are emotionally distressed, taking a ninety-minute yoga class may significantly shorten the time it takes to fall sleep and increase total sleep time.

There are many different kinds of yoga. Twenty minutes a day is a place to start. Sometimes simply centering yourself, sitting cross-legged with a straight spine and chin slightly tucked, hands in your lap or on your knees, with your palms up, can be relaxing in and of itself, without doing anything. Inhale through your nose and out through your mouth. Continue breathing and chanting a mantra (repetitive words or sound) until you feel relaxed. The chanting keeps your mind busy so that you don't go off worrying.

Many studies show that religious people are less stressed than nonbelievers. It really doesn't matter if you attend any specific church. Belief in a higher power and faith itself, of any kind, seems to make you feel more positive and contributes to relaxation and better sleep. A study at Duke University shows that religious people cope better with crises like illness, divorce, and bereavement. Religion's contribution to happiness seems almost universal across various faiths or ethnic groups. The belief in a higher power or something other than our daily reality often provides the resilience and faith we need to enjoy our lives as we age. A connectedness to things spiritual helps us overcome life's difficulties.

It is wise to trust yourself and follow your own body's unique natural rhythms, including sleep cycles. Spend time winding down in the evening. Meditate on pleasant images before sleeping, tense and release all your muscles, and make peace with the day. Reflect on all the things you are grateful for. Keep a journal of gratitude to remind yourself of what is valuable and appreciated in your life.

A calm, centered, mindfully lived life and attention to ritual and spiritual traditions are healing for many people suffering from hurry-sickness in our fast-paced world. Work on generating a peaceful way of life in your own family and social circle. Love and compassion help to create serenity.

We are always urged to have more, do more, be more, but there is a certain wise peacefulness to having enough. Slow down to a safer speed and allow yourself to enjoy your life, and take the time you need to get a good night's sleep.

Only in sleep I see their faces,
Children I played with when I was a child,
Louise comes back with her brown hair braided,
Annie with ringlets warm and wild.

Only in sleep Time is forgotten—
What may have come to them, who can know?
Yet we played last night as long ago,
And the doll-house stood at the turn of the stair.

The years had not sharpened their smooth round faces,
I met their eyes and found them mild—
Do they, too, dream of me, I wonder,
And for them am I too a child?
—Sarah Teasdale

Index